The World Health Organization

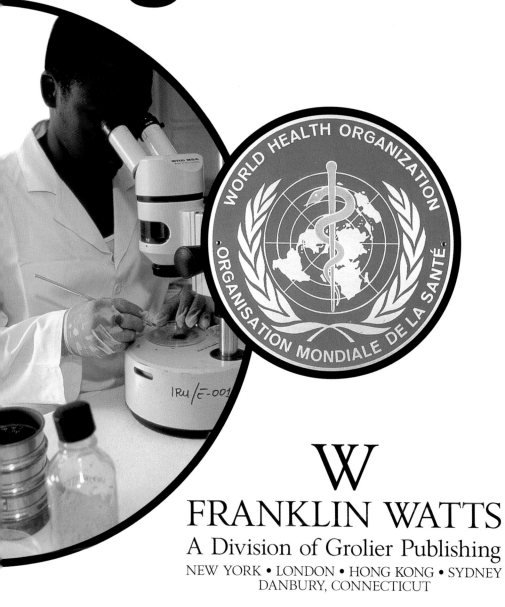

W

FRANKLIN WATTS

A Division of Grolier Publishing

NEW YORK • LONDON • HONG KONG • SYDNEY
DANBURY, CONNECTICUT

Picture credits:
Cover: WHO (copyright H. Anenden)
Inside: AKG: 7 (bottom);
Panos Pictures: 4 (bottom) 6; 13
(top); 16 (top and bottom); 17
(bottom); 18; 19 (bottom); 20
(bottom); 21; 22 (top and bottom);
23 (bottom); 24; 27 (top); 28
Rex Pictures: 27 (bottom); 29
Science Photo Library: 7 (top); 15;
19 (top). Still: 5; 14 (top and bottom) 23
(top). WHO (copyright H. Anenden): 4 (top);
8; 9; 11 (top and bottom); 12; 13 (bottom);
17 (top); 25.

Editors: Sarah Snashall, Anderley Moore
Designer: Simon Borrough
Picture research: Sue Mennell
Consultant: Gregory Hartl, WHO
Spokesperson

First published in 2000 by Franklin Watts

First American edition 2001 by
Franklin Watts
A Division of Grolier Publishing
90 Sherman Turnpike,
Danbury, CT 06816

Visit Franklin Watts on the internet at:
http://publishing.grolier.com

Cataloging-in-Publication Data is
available from the Library of Congress

ISBN   0-531-14621-9 (library bdg.)
       0-531-14815-7 (pbk.)

Printed in Malaysia

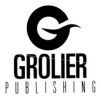

GROLIER
P U B L I S H I N G

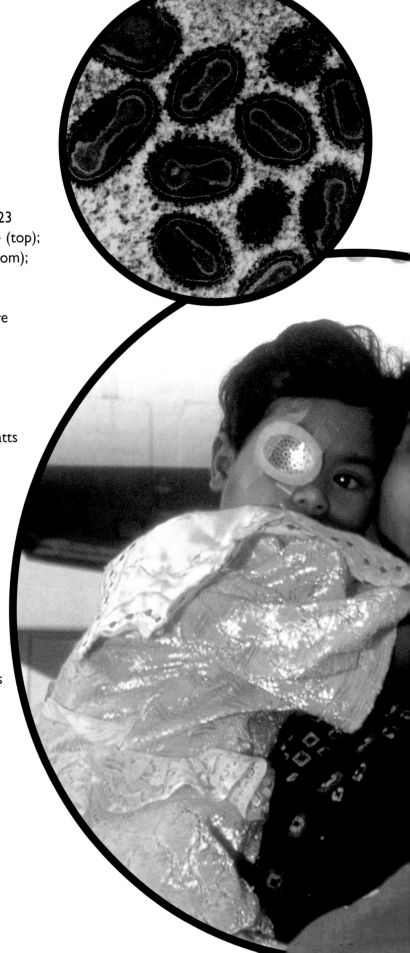

Contents

1. What is WHO?

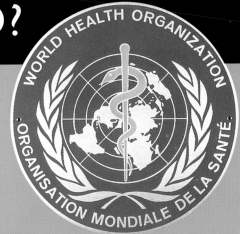

The World Health Organization (WHO) is a worldwide organization that works to bring good health to everyone in the world. It tackles global health problems such as the lack of health education and health services, and the spread of infectious and non-infectious diseases.

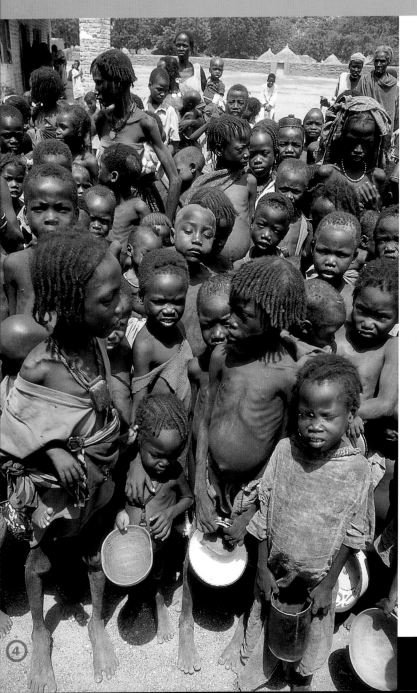

Creating World Health

WHO helps improve health for people worldwide in a number of ways. It sends health experts to train and support local health workers. It provides information and medical supplies to countries that are trying to create better health care systems. It gathers information about disease that can be used by people who are making decisions about health programs. It funds research into disease and organizes immunization programs.

 Spotlight

"Health is a state of complete physical, mental and social well-being and not merely the absence of disease or infirmity."
The World Health Organization

◀ *Malnutrition in developing countries is a growing problem as the world population increases.*

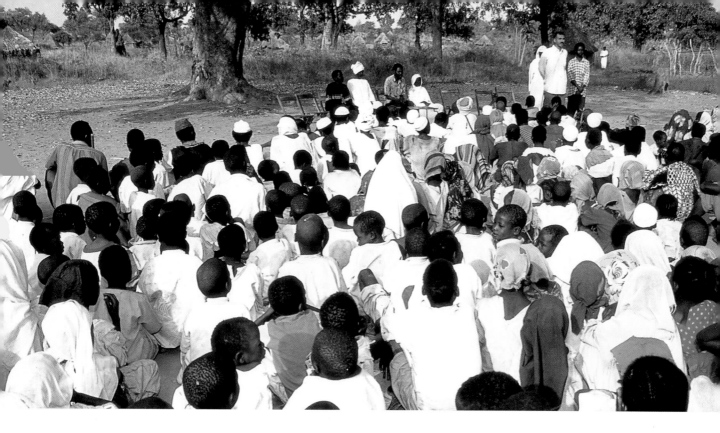

Publishing Health

WHO publishes health information in books, journals, and on the Internet. This includes training manuals, reports by experts, and the results of scientific studies funded by WHO. Information is published in six main languages: English, French, Spanish, Russian, Chinese, and Arabic.

▲ A health worker in Sudan informs villagers about drugs that can be used to fight river blindness.

▼ These Bangladeshi women are learning about clean water and sanitation.

Health Care and Diet

Many diseases, such as cancer and heart disease, can be prevented by a healthy lifestyle. In developing countries, malnutrition is caused by food shortages leading to starvation or a poor diet lacking in protein, vitamins, and minerals. In the industrialized world, malnutrition is usually caused by eating too many fatty and sugary foods and by overeating. These can lead to diseases including cancer, heart disease, and diabetes. WHO works to educate people to eat a healthy diet and to exercise regularly.

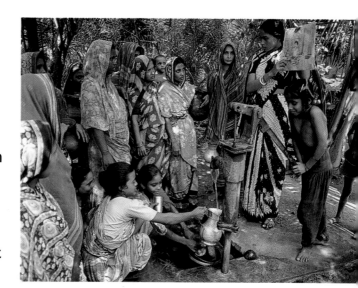

Spotlight

Tobacco Free Initiative

Every year, 4 million people die from diseases caused by smoking. WHO is working on a new international convention to control tobacco production and advertising. It works to inform and educate people on the risks of tobacco smoking. It helps member states develop anti-smoking policies such as banning tobacco advertising and introducing laws to ensure clean air for all.

▼ *A WHO field dentist checks a boy's teeth. Dental decay and gum disease are very common diseases worldwide.*

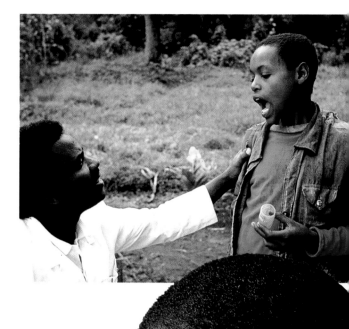

Preventing Blindness

There are about 45 million blind people in the world, and blindness is up to twenty times more common in developing countries than in the industrialized world. Two-thirds of all cases of blindness could be prevented by good nutrition and eye care. WHO helps governments set up National Blindness Prevention Programs. These programs teach people how blindness can be caused by a lack of vitamin A in the diet, and by eye infections that are not treated.

Some cases of blindness are caused by disease, such as the disease river blindness in Africa. WHO runs programs to reduce the number of blackflies that cause the disease.

▶ *A boy who has been blinded by river blindness.*

Mental Health Program

In many countries, traditional ways of life are disappearing fast. Families are breaking up, and people cannot rely on regular work or a happy home life. Many people suffer from mental illness as a result and some turn to alcohol or drugs, which harm their health. WHO estimates that about 300 million people worldwide suffer from mental illnesses.

WHO's Mental Health Program works to educate people about mental health problems, including alcohol and drug abuse.

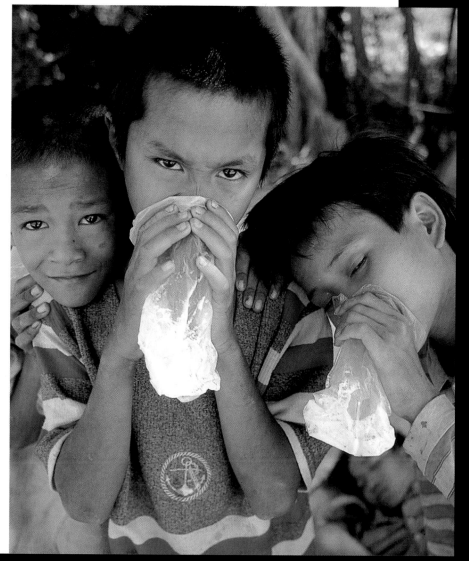

◀ *These homeless boys in Bangkok have become addicted to sniffing glue.*

One of the main tasks set out in **WHO's** constitution is to improve environmental health. This includes the food people eat, the houses they live in, the water and sanitation facilities they use, and the conditions they work in.

Problem

WHO and FAO issue guidelines and standards for food safety. Although member states are asked to accept these standards, governments can decide whether or not to make them law.

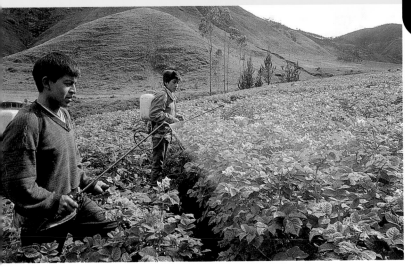

▲ *A potato crop in Peru is sprayed with pesticides.*

Food Safety

Illness caused by eating contaminated food affects millions of people each year. WHO runs a food safety program, which helps member states improve their food safety laws and systems. It works with the Food and Agriculture Organization of the United Nations (FAO) to set safe levels for pesticides and food additives.

Clean Water

One billion people in the world do not have safe drinking water — this can lead to health problems including diarrhea. WHO sets guidelines for safe drinking water and helps member states improve their water supplies.

Spotlight

In 1980, only 40 percent of people living in developing countries had access to safe drinking water, and only 20 percent had proper toilet and washing facilities. Ten years later, WHO's Program for Safe Water and Sanitation had doubled these figures.

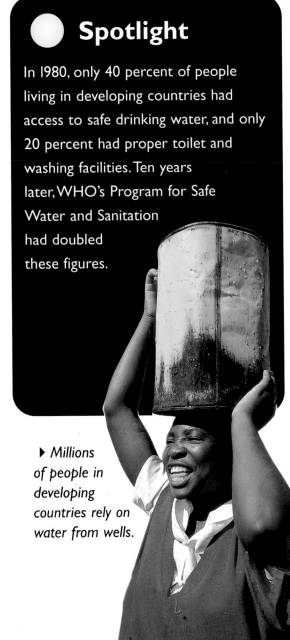

▶ *Millions of people in developing countries rely on water from wells.*

Offices of the World Health Organization:
WHO Headquarters:
World Health Organization
20 Avenue Appia
CH-1211 Geneva 27, Switzerland

WHO Regional Offices:
WHO Regional Office for Africa
(Temporary address)
Medical School, C Ward
Parirenyatwa Hospital, Mazoe Street
P.O. Box BE 773, Belvedere
Harare, Zimbabwe
www.whoafr.org

WHO Regional Office for the Americas/Pan
  American Sanitary Bureau
525 23rd Street N.W.
Washington, D.C. 20037
www.paho.org

WHO Regional Office for the Eastern
Mediterranean
P.O. Box 1517, Alexandria 21511, Egypt
www.who.sci.eg

WHO Regional Office for Europe
8, Scherfigsvej
DK-2100 Copenhagen O, Denmark
www.who.dk

WHO Regional Office for South-East Asia
World Health House
Indraprastha Estate, Mahatma Gandhi Road
New Delhi 110002, India
www.whosea.org

WHO Regional Office for the Western Pacific
P.O. Box 2932
Manila, 1000, Philippines
www.wpro.who.int

Other WHO Web Sites:
• **www.who.int**
Home page for WHO(OMS)

• **www.unsystem.org**
Directory of United Nations web sites

• **www.unaids.org**
Web site for the UN campaign against AIDS

• **www.who.int/ina-ngo**
Directory of non-governmental organizations
working officially with WHO

E-mail addresses:
• for general information on WHO, E-mail
info@who.int

• for health information, E-mail
library@who.int

• for details of publications, E-mail
publications@who.int

**Other organizations that fight against
poverty and ill health around the world:**

• Health Unlimited www.healthunlimited.org

• Health Worldwide www.healthlink.org.uk